I0420729

MIGRAINE
Natural Treatment and Prevention
The Essential Guide to Holistic Migraine Therapies

By Mary Thibodeau

Disclaimer: This book is not intended as a substitute for the medical advice of your health care practitioner. The reader should regularly consult a physician in matters relating to his/her health and diet, and particularly with respect to any symptoms that may require diagnosis or medical attention.

My Story As A Migraine Sufferer

I have had problems with headaches since I was a child, but I never had a full-blown migraine until I was twenty-eight years old. I think at some point, after years of abuse, your body will just throw you the biggest, strongest signal that something is not right. Apparently my sign was a three-day head and neck pounder, accompanied by nausea and a primal urge to completely retreat from life.

Each migraine I suffered would result in a forced fast and total cleanse, after which I would feel like a new person. But I ignored the signals and went on with my life, which included drinking gargantuan amounts of caffeinated beverages and slightly less gargantuan amounts of alcohol.

I was young and stupid and didn't spend much time worrying about what foods I ate and how much I needed to exercise. Years later those things became a priority. THE priority; because to have joy in life, and create joy for others, I believe you need a healthy body first. When I don't prioritize my health I get sick. It's pretty simple.

I finally learned that it is a bad policy to only take care of yourself when you're sick. But that's what I was doing. When the migraine came, every other part of life was shut down and I was reduced to a lump in bed with an ice bag and the shades drawn. Only when I received this enormous signal from my body was I actually getting the rest and elimination of junk that I needed.

So, what is a migraine? All of you that have experienced one can certainly describe what it feels like. Medically, when a migraine is occurring, the blood vessels in the head are rapidly dilating and become inflamed. I am able to feel the pulsating in my neck, and my shoulders, neck and head will feel very stiff and tight during these episodes. The pain is intense and often lasts from a few hours to several days.

It took me about seven years of twice-monthly migraines to figure out how to avoid them altogether. I'm hoping that someone may read this eBook and feel relief way before they've suffered through years of migraines. I've been there and I know exactly what it's like. I know that if I don't eat right, sleep, exercise and see life with gratitude, my body will send me a sign which is: "You need to upkeep that shit."

My journey to discover holistic health, which continues still, began during those first few years of migraines. Not long after my first 'real' headache, I moved to Vermont. One winter there I slipped off an icy stairway and injured my back, resulting in nerve pain that lasted for three months. While that incident remains vivid in my mind, what was even more memorable was what happened afterwards. I used a Comfrey Root compress for the first time, as suggested by my sister, to relieve the pain. The powdered up root of "Knitbone" with a bit of oil and hot water was mixed and plastered directly onto my injury. It was the only thing that made my back feel better and I could feel it working. That incident brought me to the Purple Shutter Herb shop in

Burlington for the very first time, and since then, herbs have played an ever-growing role in my life.

For years I tried various migraine medicines that were recommended by doctors, things sprayed up my nose and 'given' as suppositories, because migraine sufferers can barely hold anything down. During this time I started to get some relief during the migraines from a chiropractor that would crack my neck just right, making things start to flow easier through my head. But I was still getting them frequently and often missing work. My supervisors were concerned, because they saw what I was like during a migraine, and several co-workers suffered the same torment.

The comfrey compress had planted a seed in my brain that continues to grow. *There are other ways;* ways that recognize the body's limitations and strengths, ways that help us avoid suffering, ways that are natural with no nasty side effects. That seed led me to an herbalist, who had been a nurse at Mass General for many years and who had ultimately decided that what she was doing wasn't helping people. So she became an herbalist. I signed up to have an herbal and health consultation with her to talk about my migraines. It was she who suggested dietary changes like eliminating refined sugar and caffeine. Bingo. I haven't had a migraine as severe as the 'old days' ever since.

But I do still get some headaches. Over all these years I have figured out how to avoid them, even though I know it's not always possible. There are hormonal imbalances that can be addressed with lifestyle and nutritional changes. The lack of exercise problem seemed easy to tackle, because the rewards were so immediate and myriad.

But then there's stress, which to this day represents my final frontier of headache triggers. There are many stress reduction techniques that I enjoy and will talk about in later chapters, but in this day and age, there are times of acute stress that cannot always be avoided. For these times, having a holistic, migraine management plan comes into play by reducing the symptoms significantly.

Migraines happen for a reason and it is up to us to figure out what the problem is. Most medical practitioners will address the symptom, which to me is only a temporary fix. Even when I was taking Imitrex, supposedly the best migraine-killing drug of that time, while I did feel a reduction in head pain, I could still feel the migraine coursing throughout my body and felt absolutely terrible; my head was still throbbing only my nerves were deadened to the pain.

Throughout years of herbal and nutritional training, wildcrafting, and making herbal recipes, all the while dealing with migraines, I have learned effective ways to not only treat migraines, but to prevent them as well. I wrote this book to share with other sufferers who may be looking for relief from migraines with gentle, holistic treatments that do not cause side effects and work to eliminate the problem, not just the symptom.

Chapter 1
The Feminine Migraine:
Evening Out Hormones

About half of all female migraine sufferers have figured out over time that their headaches mainly occur according to menstrual cycles. You may find that headaches are common right before a period starts as estrogen levels are dropping, and again during ovulation when a rapid rise in the luteinising hormone (LH surge) causes more hormonal fluctuation. When I have had premenstrual migraines, I've always noticed a relief from the pain as soon as menstruation starts.

But hormones have their specific purpose in our body's design and should not, on their own, be the cause of headaches or other medical problems. Their rise and fall represents natural phases of our lives. There are many reasons why hormones may be out of balance and causing adverse symptoms. I have found that lifestyle changes can have a profound effect on hormonal headaches. Here's how:

1. Watch Iron Levels. After eating vegan for about five years, I started having problems with Anemia and from this experience I came to understand that as a menstruating woman, I need 18mg of iron every day (as opposed to 10 for men and non-menstruating women, and 30 for pregnant women). When I didn't get enough, not only were my periods heavier and more painful, but those pre-period headaches were almost guaranteed to happen at some level. As soon as I figured this out I starting making sure I got that 18mg's every day and those same relentless hormonal headaches and heavy periods have disappeared. I take a plant-based iron and B-12 supplement called Floradix every day (which is actually a beet extract with other herbs), I try to include as many greens as possible into my diet (salads, smoothies, soups) and I eat lentils regularly.

Without an iron supplement, you could have 2 cups of cooked lentils and 2 cups of steamed beet greens and more than meet that daily goal of 18mg's. I always feel it's better to get the nutrients your body needs in the form of whole organic food. But it's also good to have a natural supplement to keep meeting nutritional needs when fresh food sources aren't available or convenient.

While **beans and greens** are great sources of iron, the preponderance of processed foods in a typical American's diet has pushed these nutritional powerhouses aside for grains stripped of nutritional value, flavor enhancers, salt, refined oils and sugars. Raising the level of these two foods alone will boost iron levels and provide sources of many other vitamins and minerals. I choose lentils because they cook faster and in my experience are easier to digest than other types of legumes.

2. Stay Hydrated
I think this is key whether the headaches are hormonal or triggered by other factors. Sometimes during my worst migraines I experienced the feeling of utter dehydration, like my circulation was way too thick and viscous while my head pounded. And

during a migraine, you cannot hold down the water you need RIGHT NOW. If you have aura's, those weird feelings of imbalance and strange light visions prior to your migraine, this is the time to drink copious amounts of water. I have found that being hydrated directly prior to the migraine lessens the severity of the pain. It also, in my experience, has a positive effect on menstrual cramping and other PMS symptoms.

To stay hydrated it is essential to limit salty foods. All processed foods are salty; this is for a reason - most would taste terrible without this addictive flavor enhancer. By eating more raw fruits and vegetables, you can still get the sodium your body needs, but in a form more natural for your body to process. Added salt has no place in the life of a headache sufferer. If my period falls directly after a few days of salty restaurant meals, like when on vacation, the symptoms are inevitably worse.

You know what they say about drinking 8 glasses of water every day - this is how much our bodies need. Humans eating primarily cooked food are not getting hydrated from water rich foods like raw fruits and veggies. When I regularly get the needed amount of water everyday, I feel better in so many ways. My body seems able to handle so much more, my mood is better, and the migraines are either non-existent or manageable.

3.Magnesium
Magnesium deficiency is very common in women suffering with hormonally triggered migraines. The most common symptoms of deficiency of this mineral, such as headache, anxiety and sensitivity to

noises, match the most prevalent signs of migraines. Luckily, it is very easy to get your daily amount with whole food options. Beet Greens and Lentils again top the list of foods high in this essential mineral, while seeds, nuts and whole grains also make excellent sources.

You may hear that chocolate contains high amounts of magnesium, but because of the caffeine and the amino acid *tyramine* found in chocolate (both common triggers of migraines), I don't recommend it. But if you know that chocolate is *not* one of your triggers, then by all means, knock yourself out, and enjoy some for me while you're at it!

Every morning I have my power breakfast: an eight-banana smoothie with blueberries, which provides 80% of my magnesium (and over 100% of Vitamins C and B6). Two to three tablespoons of sunflower seeds or almonds will round out my 100% daily need.

Including dark leafy greens, beans, sweet corn, bananas, oats and small amounts of nuts and seeds every day will ensure you get enough magnesium. If you feel you cannot get your daily dose from food, many women supplement successfully with 600mg daily for migraine prevention. While the daily recommended amount of this mineral is about 300mg, studies with women supplementing with the higher dose have shown that it is safe and effective as a preventative.

4. Natural Hormonal Regulators – Soy vs. Vitex
When I mention phytoestrogens and herbs in regulating hormonal imbalance, I do not mean

suddenly including soy in every meal. Again, as a vegan, this is an easy jump to make; give up meat and embrace soy "meat" products. That is the usual course for many vegans. But soy products are very high in phytoestrogens; too high in my opinion. While I encourage people to seek out herbs and whole foods to manage imbalances, along with lifestyle changes, I would not recommend anyone to suddenly incorporate a preponderance of phyoestrogens in their diet.

Instead, I choose a gentle *all-natural* hormone regulator to work with diet, exercise and stress management. Vitex, otherwise know as Chaste Berry, represents that all natural choice, as opposed to many of the soy products available today that are far from their original source, the soy bean. Switching to soy to regulate hormones, in my opinion, is going overboard, they are too high in phytoestrogens and it is too easy to make soy products a staple in your diet.

Vitex, on the other hand, is widely known for its effects in the treatment of PMS symptoms. Since most women with migraines experience the worst headaches during PMS, numerous studies have been conducted to see the effects of hormone regulating herbs and their association with migraines.

What has been found is that Vitex can naturally regulate the level of hormones made by the pituitary gland, including estrogen and progesterone. This action effectively balances female menstrual cycles. Vitex positively reduces both the number of migraines in premenstrual women, and the duration of the symptoms. Supplementing with this herb has resulted in no adverse side effects and is well tolerated by women in studies.

Chapter 2
Migraines In Men:
Eliminating the Stigma

When my migraines were at their worst, I was working as an administrative assistant in a bank directly supporting the bank president and the senior staff. Of all the jobs I've ever had, in this one I was the most coddled. I had decided I would work in a bank while I was a restaurant manager working ungodly hours with significant stress. My only peaceful moments were crossing the street to the bank to make daily deposits. Everything at the bank seemed so serene; the employees wore nice clothes not stained with food, it was calm and quiet and everything was so organized.

A few years later, in my bank office environment, my migraine condition was *supported*. **Men are not so lucky**. I remember one of the vice presidents (a male) in the bank who also had a problem with migraines. While my co-workers went out of their way to help me get my job done so I could go home early when a migraine struck, this guy, at his peak migraine suffering, would be laying face down on his office floor, still on the phone.

I don't know where this 'migraine inequity' started, but most men cannot comfortably say, "I have a migraine" whereas women are helped and understood. Many men will go on to have their migraines misdiagnosed as a sinus headache because of this stigma. Incidentally, many sinus medications can worsen migraine symptoms. Not fair, I admit. So I feel it's time to address this discrepancy.

If men have migraines they need to have their symptoms addressed and not waived away as some unknown other problem. The facts below point to the urgency of this matter:

1.Men are at higher risk for migraines if they have played contact sports, had a concussion, or if they have had other physical trauma, or post-traumatic stress disorder.

2.When men get migraines that don't get treated, their chances of heart attacks increase.

3.Men may be less apt to seek help for their migraines because of this 'stigma'.

It's so important for men to be able to find ways of relief so that the headaches do not disrupt life and cause additional health problems. Denying or trying to ignore a migraine will only cause more stress, which makes the migraine worse.

The first step is acceptance. If one side of your head (and sometimes neck) is literally pounding, you are nauseous and/or throwing up, and any light or loud noise whatsoever is hideous to you, it's a migraine, and if you have migraines, it's time to look at the many natural techniques for prevention and treatment to improve your quality of life, and your work. So please, read on.

Chapter 3
Movement:
A Migraine Sufferer's Necessity

Fitness junkies know that the more activity you engage in, the better you feel all around. This is true at all levels of fitness. I have found that if I am walking and stretching every day, and getting in at least 2 sessions of aerobic exercise and strength training each per week, I can avoid headaches altogether. Because of the added energy, improved sleep and good feelings brought on with regular exercise, keeping all your lifestyle changes in place is easier. As soon as I slip, get too busy to exercise or feel too tired and skip my routine, my chances of headaches occurring increase. I have to prioritize and make it happen. But with steady fitness training, even low impact, my chances of migraines virtually disappear.

Important: To be clear, I do not advocate vigorous activities during a migraine!

I have tried exercising in the middle of a terrible migraine thinking, 'What the heck, it can't get any worse, and exercise always makes me feel good!' I will tell you that directly after vigorous exercise, I did feel much better – for a few minutes. But very soon after the throbbing pain came back with a vengeance. It got MUCH worse. I do not recommend vigorous exercise in the midst of a migraine. I believe a regular plan of movement, stretching and weight bearing exercise acts best as a *preventative* and not as a treatment for migraine symptoms.

Many of us have numerous things going on at once and when we are run down, it's certainly not easy to fit in exercise. As a busy Mom of three and community organizer I find what works best is exercising in 'snippets'. Even exercising for five or ten minutes can make a difference. Before I sat down to write this section, as I waited for one of my kids to get out of an activity, I decided that a 10-minute brisk walk outside would not only make me feel better, but also help me write better. Even though I felt I should work the whole time, I knew that I would work more effectively when my physical needs were met.

My loosely outlined personal regimen is this:

1-A Walk Every Day – at least 20 minutes – this is also part of my stress relief, as I walk through the woods and enjoy the peace and quiet. So usually it's a relaxing walk. If I want it to be aerobic, I simply pick up the pace, run part of it, or go hiking.

2-Aerobic Exercise – at least ½ hour, twice per week. Depending on the season, sometimes it's swimming, bike riding or rebounding, other times it's ice skating, loading wood, heavy yard work or shoveling snow (that's my ultimate favorite exercise). Once in a while I'll put in a kickboxing or zumba video. For me, changing it up is a necessary factor in sticking with my fitness goals.

3-Strength & Resistance Exercises – at least twice per week ideally.

I say ideally because a lot of times it's more like twice a month; still, a goal that I at least *try* to reach. Sometimes the quickest way for me to do this is to just get on the floor and do sets of crunches (standard, scissors, and bicycles) bridges, leg ups, etc. I tell myself to do 300 reps, and by splitting them up into sets of 40-50, I will be done in less than ten minutes. This is one of the ways I squeeze in some good exercise and I really love doing core-strengthening movements. Probably a couple times a month, sometimes less than that, I will get to my weight bench and do bench presses, dead lifts, squats, dips, etc.

There are so many options and you don't need equipment; your body can provide the weight for resistance. Choosing what you enjoy helps keep you motivated. The thing I love most about strength training is that it actually makes me feel strong – physically and emotionally.

4-Stretching – Every day. Again, there are many exercises that involve stretching and breathing, and many styles of yoga. You can take a class, or develop your own simple routine. Personally I do 10 Sun Salutations with some nice deep breathing every night before sleeping (Moon Salutations are another good option). I've done this for so many years, that even if I'm exhausted and go to bed without them, I have trouble falling sleep and end up having to get up to do them.

I always envision myself engaging in so many more fun fitness activities, only in the future, when I have more time. But for now it's essential to squeeze in what can be done to keep my body working properly. By keeping it fun, and by prioritizing the benefits of fitness, regular exercise will naturally become part of your daily routine.

Chapter 4
Finding Your Food Triggers

Trying to learn the triggers for your migraines may be a long process, but in my experience, it's well worth the effort in eliminating certain foods from the diet. The list below of common triggers is pretty exhaustive and most people will have only one or two that affect them. Mine are caffeine, chocolate (which has caffeine), refined sugar and alcohol. Taking these foods out of my diet was not that easy, and still isn't, especially the **chocolate**! Once I did though, my migraines turned back into manageable hormonal headaches and never reached the severity as when I was consuming large amounts of caffeine and sweets.

There are ways to find substitutes for your old favorites. For me, a fudge made with carob root powder mixed with some coconut oil, cashews, shredded coconut and a bit of maple syrup completely satisfies my need for something decadent, especially at family gatherings and on holidays.

None of the *non-food* triggers listed below have caused a migraine for me – but many of them certainly worsened my episodes, including flashing lights, strong odors and menstruation. Others are common triggers for many people.

There are two ways you can test for certain for migraine triggers:

1. Get tested for common allergens. An IgG food panel will test you for a hundred or more possible allergens. This type of test is for delayed hypersensitivity. In my case, once I ate chocolate or sugar, my migraine would come three days later, it was never an immediate, severe allergy. This test will help determine which foods cause your body to react with a sensitivity (slower reaction) so that you can easily figure out which foods to eliminate.

2. Track Your Habits in a Migraine Diary. Keep a journal logging daily activity, meals and snacks, and migraine occurrences and severity, for a month. Have a copy of the common migraine triggers close at hand to review during your daily journaling. Then you can refer to your log and start to see patterns with your migraines and make adjustments that way.

The migraine trigger list below outlines the most common causes with a brief explanation as to why each particular trigger can affect you and how common it is in migraine sufferers.

TRIGGERS

Tyramine
Tyramine is a chemical substance that is naturally found in many foods and certain pharmaceuticals (in particular, MAOI's). Too much tyramine can cause spikes in blood sugar and elevated hormone production, so it's best to avoid foods high in this chemical, including **aged cheese; aged, cured, pickled or smoked meats; soy products; bouillon; sauerkraut (and other fermented foods); miso soup; chocolate; fresh yeasted**

breads; red wine and beer; and dried fruit. While it may be impossible for you to avoid all these foods all the time, it's a good policy for a migraine sufferer to watch for the possible effects these foods may have on you, and try to keep these foods to a minimum.

Citrus

I have seen this listed again and again as a common migraine trigger but have not been able to find any evidence as to a reason why. Possibly, it's the fact that citrus foods are acids fruits and digest very quickly, and if you eat these types of fruits **after** a meal or on a full stomach, the fruit will be breaking down and fermenting for a while before getting digested. This may cause a blood sugar spike and/or acidity. Personally, citrus is the first food I want after a migraine has passed and I'm ready to eat again.

Coffee/Caffeinated Beverages

Research on the effects of caffeine on migraines hasn't pinpointed whether it is the caffeine itself that's the trigger, or the withdrawal from caffeine that's the big problem. But some people, who drink a lot during the week and not on the weekends, may find change in caffeine intake is a trigger for them. Certainly, any coffee hound can attest to the headaches after giving up caffeine. Either way, reducing your amounts slowly is probably the best bet for eliminating caffeine from your diet, if you think this is a trigger. Switching to green tea is a good transitioning step, as it is a healthier option and has a lower amount of caffeine per cup. Another option is to go half decaf and wean yourself down.

Nuts

I find this common trigger listed in blog post after blog post, with no apparent reason why. But other people have definitely identified nuts as a migraine trigger.

Gluten

Research has pointed to the fact that non-celiac patients, those that have a *gluten sensitivity,* are more prone to migraines than those with celiac. This sensitivity often causes inflammation of the central nervous system, which may lead to a migraine.

Onions

While studies have not been done on the onion's migraine triggering effects, there is certainly a lot of anecdotal evidence about people who got migraines after eating and/or chopping raw onions, and many point to the smell as the actual trigger.

Nitrates and Nitrites

Found in packaged meats like bacon, ham and hot dogs, **these additives are more commonly linked with migraines than any other food product**. They naturally occur in foods like celery, lettuce, beets and spinach, but it seems to be the chemical version that is used to preserve meats that is more the culprit in migraine causation.

MSG

A popular flavor enhancer and preservative, Monosodium Glutamate has shown connections with migraine symptoms since the 1960's, including severe headache, nausea and weakness, sound familiar? Studies have come back with an resounding 15% of migraines sufferers showing a sensitivity to MSG. Unfortunately eliminating this additive is quite the trick, since it has over twenty different 'aliases.' The site here gives you a rundown of all the names under which MSG may be listed in ingredient lists. MSG is found in soy sauces, marinates, seasoning packets and many other packaged foods.

Artificial Sweeteners
Aspartame (brand names are NutraSweet and Equal) can be found in about 600 products including sodas, frozen desserts, jello, gum, candy, ice cream, yogurt, drink mixes, etc. There are numerous published studies researching the negative effects of aspartame and there are over 10,000 documented cases of adverse reactions. The list of commonly reported reaction symptoms (which is very long) is topped by: *Migraines.*

Barometric Pressure
Spikes in barometric pressure or sudden weather changes are another common trigger for migraine sufferers. These changes cause fluctuations in the oxygen level and your brain's blood vessels may be doing some compensating. Some people swear by this; and that as soon as a big storm comes they feel relief.

Fasting
There are two major reasons that fasting can lead to a migraine. The first is the drop in blood sugar. The second is the release of toxins into your blood stream as you detoxify. If you feel you must fast, consider a juice fast and keep well hydrated.

Medications
This one I learned quickly; I used to take Excedrin when I first starting getting migraines and would feel better, but then it would regress and turn into a longer migraine than usual. What I didn't know then was that Excedrin has caffeine, which was one of my triggers. Common drugs that may cause 'rebound' headaches include acetaminophen, aspirin, NSAID's, MAOI's and pain medications like codeine.

Upheaval of sleep patterns – Something as small as a one-hour difference; like the twice yearly insanity that is Daylight Saving in the U.S., excluding lucky Arizonians. This time of year, in spring and fall, is always a ripe time for migraines to strike. Getting extra rest and hydration during these transitionary times is important. Also, times where your schedule suddenly changes, like going from working days to the night shift, can be a difficult time for migraine sufferers. Again, extra sleep may help here. Your body thrives with regular, substantial sleep. Migraine folk need to prioritize this.

Triggers Discussed in Previous Chapters
Menstruation
Strong odors/perfumes
Bright/flashing lights, Imax or movie theatres, strobe lights, concerts, etc.
Stress & Trauma
Dehydration

Chapter 5
Fabulous Food for Migraines

Hopefully, after reading the last chapter, you have an idea of where to start in preventing migraines by eliminating certain foods. This section is dedicated to giving you current information about which foods are actually good for migraine sufferers, in prevention and treatment. Not only will these foods help maintain a healthy, migraine ready body, most are also loaded with nutrients, fiber and water.

Greens
Most greens, especially dark leafy greens like chard, kale and spinach, are high in B2 (Riboflavin), which can have a relaxing effect on the brain, easing pain. A green juice is a great way to start your day, try 2 cups of organic mixed greens, 3 celery stalks, a bit of fresh ginger, 1 cucumber and 2 apples (add a little water if you don't have a Ninja or something similar) and blend until smooth. This mini-breakfast will net you 25% or more of B2, B5, B6; 75% of your Vitamin C, over 200% of Vitamin's K and A, and a solid amount of *every major mineral.*

Crimini Mushrooms
One cup of these mushrooms will provide over half of your daily need for Vitamin B2 (Riboflavin), plus all the other B vitamins (including a bit of B12) and a high mineral content.

Pineapples

Delicious, nutritious and sweet, pineapples have a natural enzyme that has been linked for years to pain relief. It's also an anti-inflammatory food.

Melons
High in magnesium and water content, juicy melons can help allay your headaches by addressing these deficiencies.

Carrots & Green Apples – Many times a migraine is a sign that your body is in desperate need of detoxification. Root vegetables like carrots, and green apples are high in fiber content and can help clean out the colon and give a boost to the detoxification process.

Organic Celery – Since celery is on the "Dirty Dozen" list of foods with the highest pesticide residues, I suggest buying the organic vegetable. High in luteolin, a flavanoid that can slow the inflammatory response in your brain, celery can be eaten daily to reduce the occurrence and severity of migraines.

Ginger
Make it a part of your life today. This warming herb not only tastes good, but it's a potent anti-inflammatory. Inflammation is often regarded as the root of all disease. Keep your body clean by giving it the rest, food and love it needs. Add in some ginger

Chili Peppers (Jalapenos, Habaneros) – These peppers add a delicious spicy zing to many recipes and can reduce severe pain by inhibiting a vasoactive neuropeptide that increases nerve inflammation. Just think how having a spicy soup with peppers, mushrooms, ginger, greens and celery might feel!

Chapter 6
Tips For Preventing Migraines

A few of these suggestions have been mentioned already in the previous chapters and for those, I will quickly add them in at the end of this section. I thought it would be important to have one place where all the prevention tips were located as a convenience for my readers.

Supplement with Feverfew
This highly bitter herb may not be the best tasting thing you've ever tried. In fact, if you are in the throes of a migraine it's probably not a good idea to try and eat the leaves, drink the tea, or take the tincture. But you can take the capsules if you are able to hold anything down.

For preventing migraines, take Feverfew daily (50 to 100 mg) when you *don't* have the headache. **Supplementing with Feverfew can significantly reduce the pain of migraines and their frequency.** It hasn't been established exactly how Feverfew helps migraines, but numerous studies have shown it's effectiveness.

Stress Reduction Techniques
We have to face it. This world is stressful and we have to go the extra mile and work to reduce the stress that creeps in to our daily lives. There are many ways to relieve stress, and you can choose what you like best. The most important thing here is that you choose *something* and make it a regular habit, just like exercise.

Common and effective stress relief techniques include deep breathing, meditation, yoga, singing or listening to music, positive affirmations, art therapy and many others. For me, my 'meditation' is playing the piano. When I play, I am only playing the music, no other thoughts enter my mind and I am completely relaxed and focused on the now. When I am done practicing, I feel settled and seem to have more clarity.

Chronic stress has many negative physical effects; your muscles tighten, the shoulders stiffen and your anxiety levels increase. All these effects can make migraines worse and increase their occurrences.

Earthing
For those of you that have never heard of Earthing, it's basically grounding yourself. When we are in direct contact with the earth, such as walking barefoot on the beach, we are enjoying a rich flow of electrons conducted from the earth's surface. Humans walked the earth like this long before there were shoes, carpets, cement foundations and sidewalks. By connecting with the earth directly, the increase in electrons may decrease inflammation.

While there are not any medical studies on the use of Earthing as a treatment for migraines, I was able to find personal STORIES of people who found relief using this method. If you live in a place where direct contact with the earth is impractical on a daily basis, there are Earthing sheets that can be purchased that are grounded so while you sleep, you are gaining the Earthing benefits.

Biofeedback

This method involves teaching your body to cause an influence on a particular part of your body. In the example of treating migraines, you would be taught how to affect the part of your nervous system that's in charge of blood vessel dilation. This technique can be used at the very beginning of a migraine to stop it from fully taking over. This procedure can be learned with a specialized practitioner, or you can try it yourself with the focus on relaxing your mind using the information and simple instructions in the following link:
http://www.indiana.edu/~engs/hints/hyp.htm

Avoid Over Stimulation

Sometimes a loud concert or an IMAX movie can trigger a migraine. Huge crowds, busy streets and amusement parks are examples of situations that are ripe for bombarding our senses. For migraine sufferers this may cause an episode and it's best to avoid over stimulation whenever possible.

Regular Sleep

I know this seems like a very basic no-brainer. But lack of regular sleep patterns and not enough sleep can make living a healthy lifestyle so much harder. If you want to avoid migraines, you need to be healthy. That is the whole point of the migraine – it is telling you, rather loudly, that there is a problem. Lot's of sleep, catnaps and a regular bedtime can all go so far in increasing your vitality.

Personally, when I am tired, I'm more prone to make bad food choices and am less likely to exercise. In a nutshell, I have to sleep to stay healthy and avoid migraines. To me, adequate sleep means nine hours every night.

Live in the Moment
I would hazard a guess that many migraine sufferers are over achievers. They have a millions things on their plate at once and never slow down. Others may have an incredible amount of stress in their life. Either way, living in the present can lessen the stress that often brings about or worsens a migraine.

Coenzyme Q10
This vitamin-like substance that is in almost every cell of our body, works to protect and maintains cells, aids in digestion and acts as a powerful antioxidant. While data doesn't point to exactly why taking extra Coenzyme Q10 reduces migraines, the studies reveal that overwhelmingly, the pain, symptoms, severity and frequency are reduced with supplementation.

Prevention Techniques Discussed In Previous Chapters:
Regular Exercise – Stretching, Aerobic and Strength Training
Anti-Inflammatory Diet
Addressing Hormonal Imbalance
Keeping Properly Hydrated - 8 cups per day

Chapter 7
Symptom Relief

It is my hope that this book will provide enough information so that you have options for prevention methods and eventually live migraine free. Until you get to that point it's essential to have many gentle and toxin-free ways of relieving the migraine once you are in it. For all of you sufferers out there, maybe you have found something that works for you. Below I will outline the tips that have helped me endure the very worst of my migraines, in order of what worked absolutely best for me and so on.

Chiropractic Care
When my migraines were happening regularly about every two weeks, I was lucky to have found a young Chiropractor who would take me on short notice as she was still building up her business. I think her 'bedside' manner was what made the whole process effective. She was kind and soft spoken, and genuinely seemed concerned about me.

As an aside, I once went to a Chiropractor who was new in town, and on his waiting room wall was an enormous painting depicting a golf course with well-dressed Caucasian golf players having a grand old time while the African American caddies and servants were sweating it out and looking harried. I thought it a very racist depiction and already had a negative first impression of this Chiropractor before I went into his office. Of course mentioning the painting upon meeting him was probably not the best way to start but I couldn't help myself.

Anyway after this discussion, he proceeded to check me over but his manner was so rude and condescending and I ended up walking out of there. My point in all this is that you have to be at ease with your practitioner if healing is going to take place. If you're stressed by simply being in the presence of someone or you find the office environment hostile in anyway, it's best to find another.

So back to the lovely Dr. D. She would try to relax me a bit, massaging my shoulders and having me do some gentle neck exercises and then would give me this neck crack that would give me immediate relief. I could feel my circulation improving; like something had loosened and was a draining. I would go home, go to sleep and wake up feeling like a new person. It took some time but immediately after her care I could feel the difference, and I knew it was getting better. This simple knowledge helped speed up the process, since the stress of having the headache for three days (and the loss of work hours and life that went along with it) seemingly made the migraines worse.

Ice
I was practically in love with my ice bag in those days. A large, cotton flannelled, hand sewn bag filled with rice that I kept in the freezer was my only friend during a migraine. I would lie on the side where the pounding was the worst with the bag under my neck and close my eyes to the world. It definitely brought relief. I would even recommend having two so they can be rotated and you don't have to go without. This would make a thoughtful gift for any migraine sufferer in your life.

Feverfew/Chamomile Tea
This is only recommended when migraine sufferers
are able to hold liquids down. In my experience, the
feverfew eliminates the nausea and the chamomile
is a calming sedative and a powerful anti-
inflammatory. You could drink this (or supplement
with tinctures or capsules) every day as a
preventative as well.

Lavender Essential Oil
I used so much of this calming, nausea-reducing
herb during my migraine stage, that for a long time
after the migraines went away, I had a negative
association with it. After the worst of my migraines
were out of my life, the smell of lavender essential
oil would remind me all too much of how I felt
when I had a migraine, and for a period of time, I
had an aversion to it, not wanting at all to be
reminded of that suffering. I have gone back to
using it in homemade herbal products and home
cleaners but I have certainly lost that tight affinity
with it that I once had.

But during a migraine, even the worst pounders, the
essential oil of this powerful herb would help relax
me and relieve the nausea. I would put drops on my
pillow or take a bath with 10-20 drops in it.
Inhalation of the vapors of this herb can directly
curtail the symptoms of a migraine by acting as a
natural analgesic, sedative, nervine and
antispasmodic.

Sleeping in Darkness
After years of migraines, I started to wonder if I
simply made sure I got enough sleep all the time

maybe I could avoid them altogether. I still think this may be a valid strategy. I believe that migraines happen when your body has 'had it'. Between the food we eat, the stress we are faced with and the lack of sleep, maybe extra rest is all we need. Could the headache that would reduce me to a lump in bed for up to three days be avoided by having enough rest in the first place? Definitely something to ponder.

But whether your body needed rest before your migraine or not, you will definitely need it *during* the migraine. If you are a migraine sufferer I probably do not have to tell you this – when you are in the throes of the headache, if you are not in bed, surely you are wishing desperately to be there.

If it stresses you out to miss work or other life events, remember that stress can make your migraine worse and rest can help you feel better. You've got to take care of yourself now.

Happy Thoughts
If you have a migraine right now you are probably swearing at me and thinking what a bunch of bunk! But while you are resting with your migraine (which you should be), instead of thinking about all the deadlines you are missing, all the disappointments you may have caused or all the schedules you have had to change, try focusing on gratitude. Just try to start a list of all the things for which you are truly thankful. Thoughts like these actually have positive effects on your body, physically and emotionally. Dwelling on all the problems caused by your migraine does nothing to

help your situation. Thinking about what you love in your life, and how lucky you are, will.

Chapter 8
Can Marijuana Eliminate Migraines?

Though the laws for medical use of marijuana throughout the U.S. vary, twenty-three states have now legalized this herb for use in certain conditions, and a few states have even legalized it for recreational use.

In Maine, marijuana may be used in cases of certain diseases including cancer, glaucoma, HIV and Alzheimer's, or for specific symptoms like seizures, severe nausea, severe muscle spasms and chronic or intractable pain (intractable pain includes pain that hasn't been relieved after six months of standard treatment). It certainly seems to me that migraines fit in with these requirements, between the chronic pain and nausea. I have not personally sought a prescription because I have found other ways to deal with my migraines, but I feel that this herb surely is a solid possibility to treating migraines and well worth discussing with your health care practitioner.

A study in the 1980's tracked the health of longterm marijuana users after they abruptly stopped smoking. The patients developed migraines shortly after eliminating this herb. The theory was that after the patients stopped smoking they no longer were producing the natural pain relieving chemicals in their brains. Human brains have their own analgesic neurochemicals that are naturally occurring and can prevent or reduce the pain of a migraine. These chemicals can be stimulated by triptans (often seen in migraine pharmaceuticals) and marijuana. Once the drug was no longer taken, the chemicals were no longer being stimulated enough for migraine avoidance, at least that is the theory.

The standardization and federal regulation of any herb is a wildcrafter's nightmare. I would rather leave the herb growing to gardeners and not see pharmaceutical companies getting involved with producing 'extraction' products like Marinol, where certain properties are extracted for their power in relieving a certain symptom.

It's my preference with medicine in general to use nature's medicine in the form of whole plants. The only good news I can think of about government regulation is that more and more studies are being funded meaning more information will be available as legalization proliferates the need for further research.

People have long been using marijuana as a medicinal herb but only recently, since legalization, has an interest in the studies of its effects grown. While scientific studies are far and few between, anecdotal evidence is abound. What we know through the information we do have and through personal use (over 3,000,000 Americans smoke pot every day) is this:

Marijuana relieves stress and anxiety, is calming, pain relieving and quite possibly cancer fighting. We know that people with Glaucoma, Hepatitis C, HIV, Cancer, Crohn's Disease, Arthritis, MS, IBS, seizure disorders and chronic pain or nausea have found relief from their symptoms (and at times increased health) while taking this herb.

And though marijuana has some side effects including dry mouth and eyes, increased appetite, lessened coordination, increased heart rate, apathy, mood swings and proneness to bronchial issues (when the herb is smoked), this 'drug' has never once caused a death. Compare this list to the side effects of Imitrex: mild headache, pain or chest tightness, heavy feeling or pressure in any part of your body, weakness, feeling hot or cold, spinning sensation, dizziness, drowsiness, nausea, vomiting, drooling, bad taste in mouth, burning or irritation in nose, and warmth, redness or tingling under the skin. After I read these I was then directed to the website for a comprehensive (!) view of information on its side effects.

Note: By making teas or 'baked' goods with marijuana, or by using a vaporizer, you can negate any lung problems that smoking may cause.

As an herbalist I feel like I would be remiss in leaving out marijuana as a viable herb in treating and/or preventing migraines. By looking at the specific properties in relation to migraine symptoms I can see how this plant would help:

1. Analgesic – pain relieving is so important when you have a migraine.

2. Anti-Anxiety – feeling the stress and anxiety of the migraine in my opinion is probably the worst part; marijuana has long proven anti-anxiety properties.

3. Anti-Nausea – if you are too nauseous to eat and drink, marijuana has been shown repeatedly to reduce this symptom. This has a domino effect, once you are able to eat and hold down water, you will feel better cumulatively.

4. Appetite Stimulating – this goes along with the anti-nausea; if you have been unable to eat due to nausea and pain, this herb helps with increasing your appetite so you can get those needed nutrients.

Bonus Chapter
I Had A Migraine Today: Here's Why

After all of these years of preventing and treating migraines, I still get one occasionally. Earlier this week I went to a birthday party for my friend's little daughter. She had made a gorgeous apple crisp with fresh picked apples, coconut oil and other gluten free ingredients. And sugar. I asked her what sweetener she used so I knew up front. I thought, "Just one bite won't hurt!" It is amazing how the mind can force the body to forget – I just wanted to be social and taste something yummy. It was only one bite, though rather large, and sure enough, exactly three days later, I started having the signs.
In my defense, I had successfully avoided all refined sugar for over a year.

Last night, as I sat in a gym with a couple hundred other people and kids for cross-country awards after my daughter's meet, I knew for sure it was acoming. Yep, really, *one* bite of apple crisp with refined sugar in it was enough to trigger my migraine. I knew it while driving to the meet when the rain pattering on the roof of my car felt bothersome, and I wasn't cranking tunes during one of my only child-free moments of the day.

I tossed and turned all night with the neck and head pain developing and frequent trips to the freezer to trade out ice bags. Before bed, I had made a strong chamomile/feverfew tea and sipped on that during the night, and made sure yesterday to drink a lot of liquids. This morning I wasn't what you would call bright and chipper as I helped kids off to school and homeschooled one. But I was functional. Later in the morning I took a long shower and a nap before going to school conferences. In the afternoon it was a bit hard to avoid stress, a migraine must, as I was asked to helped my soon-to-be-ex install a gas stove, 'together.' The migraine got worse and after a bit I excused myself for another nap with ice.

Today was my day to get a million things done. Some of the projects I had slated for the day included marketing work in my publishing business, finding a place to live, securing part-time, work-from-home jobs, working on my non-profits, and gads of housework. But I was able to push it all aside until the weekend, and there was only a teensy thought about, "What if the migraine lasts three days?!" Then I would be totally screwed. But I kept my thoughts on this book and everything I had learned over the years.

Keep hydrated, take feverfew and chamomile, take good, good care of myself with rest and long hot showers. Smile inwardly and force myself to list reasons why I am grateful. Be in the moment. Cut myself a huge slice of slack. And you know what? It's only the second day and the migraine is but a mere thump on the side of my neck and head. I'm pretty confident that I will be like new tomorrow morning. No nausea, no vomiting and the pain is probably at a '3'. My migraines at my worst had me down and out for three straight days, vomiting all of one day, nauseous for two, and the pain at an eight or higher.

With lifestyle choices I can cut down drastically on the occurrences of migraines, and with holistic, herbal and relaxing treatments, I can reduce their severity. I feel very thankful to have learned my migraine triggers and ways to make the symptoms liveable, and I only hope that my readers do not have to suffer for years before they figure out their own plan for migraine treatment. I do hope that the suggestions and practical life experiences I have shared with you in this book help you to do just that.

I have been a good mom and am giving and patient with my kids. When I have a migraine they tend to be very helpful and understanding, even though none of them get headaches at all (thankfully!). But they see all that I do and the pressure I am under and they know sometimes I absolutely need to rest and take care of myself. This was much harder when they were little, but back then, their needs came first no matter what. And because those needs were met when they were younger (and that's another book!), they are now able to handle a mom that might suddenly need to just lay down for an afternoon.

(The next day after my very last migraine)...Last night, I slept for twelve - that's right - twelve hours last night and I did indeed wake up feeling like a new person. I got the rest and care my body needed and the headache was gone during the night. I am still drinking some feverfew and ginger tea, because it just feels good to do so. I got outside this morning and worked on getting some video and photos for my next book about tree medicine. Got caught up on laundry, baked two apple pies for the kids and worked enough to erase that overwhelmed feeling.

During the past week, I had exercised plenty. I walked every day for at least twenty minutes. One day I did 300 reps of crunches and bridges and on two separate days I loaded wood for at least an hour. Every night I did my ten sun poses before bed. My diet, other than the fateful spoonful of apple crisp, was plant based with plenty of fruit and vegetables and regular meal times. I made sure to take my iron and B12. Though it was a busy week, I tried my best to keep healthy habits going strong and the result was a migraine that was manageable and lasted only one full day, as opposed to three.

I think many people have way too much stress in their lives and maybe what is needed is to just to do a lot more of "nothing" or "laying around resting" so that a migraine doesn't come along and force the issue. Migraines offer the supreme reminder to take it easy, slow down and care for our selves. Sometimes the only way I have survived migraines is by viewing them as a gift - a very potent message to look closely at my life and stop ignoring my needs.

Conclusion
You Have the Power to Improve Your Health

I remember when my migraines started, at the time my work schedule was insanely stressful. Some days I worked at 5am until 4pm. Other days I worked from 4pm to 2am. During all hours of the day I was ingesting caffeine at a frightening rate to keep going. The place where I worked was a coffee house and restaurant that seated 250 people and was busy all the time, as it was situated on the campus of ASU. Only the best and freshest ingredients were used in all their drinks, food and desserts and they encouraged employees to sample freely in order to make recommendations. I started drinking iced cappuccinos by mixing about 1/8 espresso with 7/8 milk. After a few months, I was filling the large iced cup with espresso and adding only a splash of milk. I was sucking down iced café mochas like crazy as well, the most heavenly delicious drink ever known to me, topped with whipped cream and cinnamon.

So do I miss the iced café mochas? Yes I do. I can taste one right now. Do I miss a lovely sombrero with coffee brandy and milk? Of course! And do I miss having a slice of chocolate cake or a few chocolate chip cookies or a strawberry cheesecake ice cream cone? Yes, yes and yes. Sugar, caffeine and chocolate do not agree with my body and though I remember them fondly, I'm O.K. with going without for the better good of me. No migraine is worth a latte. With so many good things in my life, I don't need any of these 'goodies'. Though I'll admit, when I can get a good cup of decaf coffee, it does feel like a treat.

I want to end my book by telling you about my daughter and her miracle dress. A few years back, at age seven, she was gearing up for Halloween and we had bought her a beautiful princess dress with tiara, matching shoes and spangly jewels. The night before Halloween, she came down with a high fever and was up during the night with body aches and general miserableness.

When she woke up on Halloween morning she was still running a fever and was lethargic and did not want any food. I had 'the talk' with her about missing trick or treating later that night and with that sudden realization, she got up, went into her room and put on her dress and accessories. When she came out an hour later, I swear her fever was gone and she went on to eat a hearty breakfast and play outside with her brothers.

I watched her that whole day and she literally was fine. She had willed herself to be better so she could go out trick or treating in her grandparents' neighborhood, where everybody decorated and many people even had haunted houses in their garage. She went trick or treating (back then we had the candy fairy who gave cash and organic candy in return for their spoils), and even the next day, the sickness was gone. We dubbed that *The Day of the Miracle Dress.*

Why am I bringing this up? Because to me this is perfect example of how we can affect our own health. Not just what we eat, but what we tell ourselves, what we decide about how we are going to react during a sickness. With a migraine, you have to put on your miracle dress (or miracle pants) and tell yourself it's going to be O.K. Don't give into the stress – instead, make the best of your life, look inward, take care and change your health naturally. We have the power; it's just a matter of calling it up.

Thank you so much for reading and I truly hope it helped you find a solution to your migraines. Please leave a review when done reading; it really helps with the book's ranking to have reviews, whether you liked the book or not!

To receive my free eBook:
"Ten Wild Herbs For Ten Modern Problems",
go to www.boondocksbotanical.com.

Other books by Mary Thibodeau:
"Vegan: How To Be A Vegan In A Meat Eater's World" Available at Amazon.com

Free Bonus eBook:

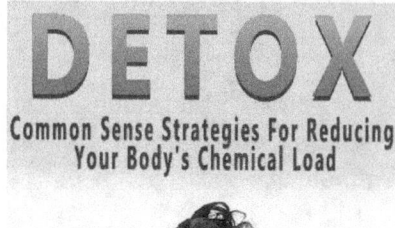

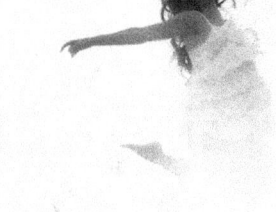

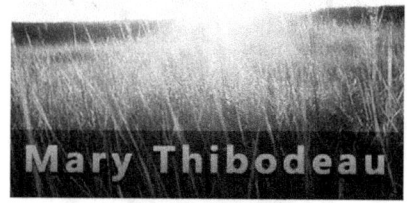

DETOX:
Holistic Strategies
For Reducing Your
Body's Chemical Load

substitute for the medical advice of your health care practitioner. The reader should regularly consult a physician in matters relating to his/her health and diet, and particularly with respect to any symptoms that may require diagnosis or medical attention.

Table of Contents

Introduction
What's Ailing Us?

While the rates of sickness and disease in the United States continue to rise faster than our population growth, facing health issues with clear directives becomes increasingly important. We have more food, more doctors, and certainly more information than ever – yet the people of our country and those that follow our lead continually get sicker.

Hunger in the United States has taken on a unexpected face. While food is abundant, the supply available to our families is alarmingly devoid of nutrients. We are not in need of calories, because we get plenty, but we are hungry for the foods our bodies need. Not only are commercial foods lacking in minerals, vitamins and fiber, but they are also filled with artificial colors and flavors, non-human hormones, antibiotics, and a myriad of 'non-food' additives. The highly processed and heavily marketed foods sold in our supermarkets ensure optimal profits for food producers and substandard nutrition for its consumers.

In 1980 the U.S. population was approximately 227,000,000 with the number of doctors at 467,679. Thirty years later the population had grown to 309,000,000 and the number of doctors reached 985,375 ("Total Number Of Doctors", 2010). While the number of physicians during that time grew at a rate of 53%, the population increased by only 27% ("Historical Population", 2015). In my own hometown, since the 1980's, the proliferation of new doctors' offices and 'health malls' has dominated commercial development while the population has remained basically the same.

During this same era, cancer rates in children ages 0-19 rose from 15.6 per 100,000 kids in 1980 to 17.3% in 2010. This trend continues to increase as data from 2014 shows that rate is up to 21.1%. The average age of a child with cancer is six and in 2013 alone, 58% of all child deaths were caused by cancer. One child out of every eight will not survive their bout with cancer. For adults, one out of every two men in the U.S. will have cancer at some point, while two out of every three women will be afflicted ("Cancer and your Environment", 2012).

How do we account for the fact that we have a reliable food supply and an excessively large medical establishment but our rates of sickness continue to grow? It has been ingrained in our minds that a healthy lifestyle with a plant-focused diet, regular exercise and stress management can reduce the rates of cancer, heart disease, obesity, diabetes and many of the other diseases that plague our nation. But can we say in all certainty that exercising, reducing stress and eating healthy is enough?

What This Book Does For You
Our bodies our literally inundated with toxic chemicals from all angles of life. From the food we eat and the drugs we take, to the water we drink and the air we breathe, toxins now threaten our health on a wide spectrum basis. In this book we will look closely at the major sources of common toxins that

find their way into our bodies and discover strategies to avoid their ill effects as much as possible to support our inner vibrancy.

Chapter One
Toxins In The Commercial Food Supply

It's very difficult to face the reality of our toxic food supply. But by taking a close look at what toxins we are ingesting during our meals, and by understanding ingredient lists and available options, we gain so much power in affecting our health. Regulating what's going into our bodies three or more time per day is by far the fastest and most efficient way to clean up our inner environment.

The amount of chemicals now entering our digestive tracts everyday through our food supply is mind-boggling. Synthetic hormones, artificial flavors and colors, flavor enhancers, 'enriched' flours and highly processed fats have thoroughly invaded the ingredient lists of grocery store items. Labeling laws are deceptive and inadequate at best and benefit food sellers, not consumers. When you see *'all natural ingredients'* on a food package it means essentially nothing. According to the FDA, this term is not clearly defined or regulated. It is assumed that 'all natural' products do not include any artificial ingredients, but only meat and dairy items labeled 'all natural' are *ever checked* ("What Is The Meaning Of Natural", 2015).

Natural flavors, found in most packaged foods, are originally derived from a plant or animal but are usually highly processed, chemically extracted substances that in no way resemble their original food source. Their chief function is not nutritional, but only to add flavor and reduce costs for the seller. Such 'flavors' include extracts of fish bladders, anal secretions of beavers and solutions of crushed beetles - probably not what you want to see when reading your breakfast cereal ingredients. That's why they are all lumped under the 'natural flavor' category.

There are **thousands** of food additives, natural and synthetic, that are regularly used in our foods, including things like '*Diethylenetriamine crosslinked with epichlorohydrin*' (I read 3 different explanations of this item and still have no idea what it is), and '*Erythromycin*', an antibiotic that's derived from uncooked tissues of chickens, turkeys and beef cattle. Having a close look at this list is quite frightening. What's being done to our food? What **are** we eating?

Before these foods even get a chance to have 'natural' ingredients added in, they have already been subjected to many stages of chemical exposure. Pesticides, including herbicides, insecticides and fungicides, represent the group of chemicals used to kill undesirable organisms. Though the EPA regulates pesticide residues and encourages less toxic chemicals and non-toxic pest control methods, they do not regulate how many different pesticides can be used, nor do they limit the sum of residues from all the contaminants.

Atrazine is one of the most common pesticides used in the U.S., with over _80,000,000 pounds_ being applied annually, mostly on corn crops in the mid-west. While the EPA maintains the safety of this product, several studies have linked Atrazine to birth defects, infertility and cancer. Residual amounts of Atrazine are in our food supply and in one study were found to have contaminated 100% of the groundwater sites studied. It has been estimated that between 4,000 and 20,000 cancer cases per year are caused by the residue of this one pesticide ("H.R. 2044", 2013).

There are currently over 1200 different pesticides registered for use in America.
Their sales in the U.S. during the year 2007 totaled $12,454,000,000 ("Pesticides Industry Sales and Usage", 2007). In my region, where 'wild' blueberries are regularly sprayed, there are 16 listed pesticides that may be used. One of them is highly toxic to humans, five are moderately toxic to humans, and almost all of them are categorized as highly toxic to bees and fish. Incidentally, the pesticide approved for wild blueberries in Maine that is highly toxic to humans (as well as bees and fish) is also listed as only 'slightly' effective ("2014 Maine Wild Blueberry Pesticide Chart", 2014).

Holistic Strategies
For Limiting Toxic Chemicals In Our Food

Buy Organic Foods
Organic produce and cereals have been shown repeatedly to not only contain less pesticide residues, but they also provide significantly higher levels of antioxidants (Mosbergen, 2014). Choosing organic foods may be cost-inhibitive to some, but

buying in bulk or through natural food co-ops can help allay the expense of buying organic.

Grow Your Own Food
This is the one way you can be sure of exactly what is put into your food supply. The benefits are exponential, as when you garden, you experience more fresh air, get more exercise and become more connected to your food. Perhaps the biggest benefit of gardening is the ability to have fresh picked produce on your plate. No shipping, storing or packaging necessary. For those in metropolitan areas or with limited garden space, vertical gardening may be a helpful option.

Limit Or Eliminate Foods With Highest Pesticide Residues
If you cannot afford to buy your food organically, you have the option to avoid foods listed as having the highest residual toxins:

Non-Organic Foods to Avoid
Peach
Apple
Sweet Bell Pepper
Celery
Nectarine
Strawberry
Cherry
Pear
Imported Grape
Spinach
Lettuce
Potatoes
("The Dirty Dozen", 2015)

It may seem that all your favorite produce items grace this list, but fortunately these 'dirty dozen' compilations have been out for years and these foods are often sold organically. My local supermarket currently offers eight of these items in organic versions. Many of these foods are also easily grown at home.

Additionally, there's a list for foods at the bottom of the scale of pesticide residuals. Incorporating more of these foods while eliminating items from the 'dirty dozen' list can help reduce your toxic exposure.

<u>Non-Organic Foods With Lowest Amount Of Toxic Residuals</u>
Onion
Avocado
Sweet Corn (frozen)
Pineapple
Mango
Asparagus
Sweet Peas (frozen)
Kiwi
Banana
Cabbage
Broccoli
Cauliflower
Eggplant
Grapefruit
Cantaloupe (domestic)
Sweet Potato

Chapter Two
Pharmaceuticals And The
'Take A Pill' Mentality

In the United States we have, as a society, chosen convenience over health. Instead of adjusting our lifestyle to emphasize exercise, healthy foods, stress management and adequate sleep, we have shown our preference to taking a pill to reduce the symptoms of unhealthy living.

This is not an easy habit to reverse. The profit margins of drug manufacturers are the highest of any other industry, even outweighing banking, oil companies and the media. As a result, the drug industry is able to pay billions of dollars promoting their products. In 2013 alone, Johnson & Johnson spent $17.5 billion on sales and marketing (Swanson, 2015). This is no surprise to anyone watching prime time TV or perusing the internet, where drug ads are pervasive. Pharmaceuticals can afford the best marketers and attorneys, and can also afford the fines for falsely promoting drugs that haven't been yet approved.

Drugs are far more commonplace in society than ever. Standard summer camp forms for kids now leave out a ¼ page for information about a child's prescriptions, as though it is perfectly normal for kids to be on multiple medications. This new normal shows acceptance for the premise that even our kids don't need to live healthy lifestyles when all they have to do is take pills to reduce their symptoms. They are becoming dependent on pharmaceuticals to suppress symptoms of disease. These pills to not cure sickness. They simply muffle the human body's system of signaling that something is wrong.

Not only have we come to depend on prescriptions and over-the-counter medicines to mask our illnesses; we have become lazy about reading their labels. Consumers and their health care practitioners largely ignore the lists of adverse reactions and side effects. Whether the ingredient is active or non-active, it is a synthetic chemical that likely has negative effects on the body.

Before the age of six months, each infant in the United States will have received 20 or more vaccines (up from 10 in 1983). It's not even so much the active disease that is injected into the bloodstream of infants, but the other ingredients that are a cause of concern. Formaldehyde and Aluminum Phosphate top the list on the ingredient disclosures for vaccines. According to the CDC's public website, formaldehyde causes some cancers when breathed in environmentally. I personally have a hard time believing that repeated formaldehyde injections have no detrimental effects, yet according to the FDA, small amounts over time have not been linked to cancer like the environmental form. The process of having 49 vaccines during a person's years of formation does not make a whole lot of sense to me. Maybe I'm as crazy as vaccine supporters think I am - maybe not. While the safety of vaccines is forcefully shoved down the throats of Americans, studies verifying the safety of the cumulative effects of all the combined vaccines remain non-existent. Meanwhile, one drug company alone (Merck) was able to reap $17.1 billion in profits in 2014 ("Company Fact Sheet", 2015).

Holistic Strategies
For Limiting Pharmaceuticals

Make Lifestyle Changes a Priority
We hear this again and again. Lifestyle changes. Why do we have to change? Some people find it difficult to alter their habits but I think this may be due to lack of energy because of those very same habits. But in my experience, lifestyle changes WORK. Instead of using steroidal creams to suppress my eczema, I switched out wheat and added in organic spelt. Eczema gone. For migraines, instead of taking Imitrix, Excedrin, Naproxin or any of the 81 other common migraine drugs available, I gave up caffeine and white sugar. Instead of heaping drug interactions and side effects onto a body that was already screaming for relief, I made an adjustment to my lifestyle that not only removed those 3-days migraines, but made me healthier overall in the long run.

Tell your healthcare practitioner you are interested in making lifestyle changes to improve your health and limit your dependence on prescriptions. If they are not interested in working with you on this, find someone new.

What are some of the changes you can make to reduce the amount of pharmaceuticals in your body? You know them already: Get more sleep, incorporate stress reduction techniques like deep breathing or yoga, eat more plant-based foods and exercise.

Support Your Liver
For people that are on multiple medications daily, it is important to find help for an overtaxed liver. No bodily organ was designed to handle the toxic load we create by taking pills every day.

1. Supplement With Milk Thistle
This gentle, naturally detoxifying herb has been used for centuries in treating liver ailments. Containing Silymarin, a substance shown to protect the liver from toxins and support liver cell repair, a daily supplement of Milk Thistle will aid in overall liver health.

2. Keep Hydrated
A dehydrated system will simply hinder the removal of toxins. Drinking plenty of filtered water each day will encourage your liver to do its job of flushing out waste chemicals.

3. Include foods that are naturally good for your liver, like Grapefruit
A large glass of fresh squeezed grapefruit juice each morning is a great way to support your liver. With its high content of Vitamin C and liver enzyme boosting capability, this delicious drink helps your liver by encouraging the flushing out of toxins. Other liver-supporting foods include leafy greens, which neutralize heavy metals and other harmful chemicals in the bloodstream; and beets and carrots, which contain properties that stimulate healthy liver detoxification.

Chapter Three - Bodycare Products: What Chemicals Are We Putting On and In Our Bodies?

The third way in which toxins commonly work their way into our life is hidden in the body care products we use. By applying commercial make-up, creams, lotions, shampoos, soaps, deodorants and sunscreens, we might feel like we're taking good care of our appearance or nurturing our skin. In reality we are embracing an unprecedented intake of foreign substances through our largest organ. Those of you who were disheartened to read the summary of food additives in Chapter 1 will not be happy to know that the list of chemicals available for use in body care products currently tops 150,000 ("Skin Deep", 2015).

Many of the more common ingredients are known carcinogens and/or hormone disruptors, while some are listed as pesticides. Artificial colors derived from coal tar, a recognized carcinogen to humans, is found in make-up and hair dyes, while Phthalates are often disguised as 'fragrance' in the ingredient lists because of their known toxicity to the reproductive system ("Why This Matters", 2011). For many years, those with allergies and respiratory disease have been avoiding these products, for good reason. Chemicals like sodium lauryl sulfate, which is found in most body care products, has been found to cause skin and eye irritations and respiratory problems.

Since Westerners average nine different body care products per day, reducing their use or switching to homemade and organic products will significantly reduce the number of toxins taken in daily.

Holistic Strategies
For Limiting Commercial,
Toxin-Heavy Body Care Products

Make Your Own Natural Body Care Products
This may seem daunting but with a few ingredients found in natural food stores, many regular supermarkets and even your own kitchen, you can make shampoo, make-up and just about any skin or body care treatment you need. Noxema, (which to me, even *sounds* like a disease) sells make-up removal cloths that feature Triclosan as its active ingredient. Triclosan is an antibacterial agent that has been shown to affect hormonal regulation. You could buy those and apply them directly to your face and EYES every night to remove make-up, or you could use Coconut Oil, which will remove your make-up and moisturize gently without toxins. Click here to be taken to a beautiful eBook by my friend Carmen Reeves. It's full of recipes to make your own organic, cruelty-free products and make-up. You can spend less to make your own, and have a better quality, toxin-free product.

Buy Organic
If you don't have the time or inclination to make your own bodycare products, purchasing organic items makes a great choice. While organic often means more expensive, these products have been shown to cause fewer allergic reactions and skin

irritations and, in my opinion, they have a much more pleasing scent.

Simplify

Why do we need ten or more body care products every day anyway? Are we that hideous? Honestly, I have not worn make-up or deodorant in over a decade. I am a true believer that beauty comes from within, and that bad smells are the result of unhealthful living habits or stress. Yes, we all have a body odor and that is natural. This mentality is not always easy to maintain in our commercially driven world and it becomes the choice of each individual what they put on their body, in their hair or all over their face. Limiting body care products will allow us to limit our chemical exposure and save money.

Try Shea Butter

Another way to reduce toxins going into our skin is to reduce ingredients. By using 100% pure Shea Butter you are rewarded with a high quality, non-toxic and luxurious-feeling moisturizer. It has no fragrance, is cruelty-free, and a little goes a long way. It's also effective in treating dry skin conditions, eczema and psoriasis. A 7oz. (207ml) tub of Shea Butter can be bought for about $10.00 at most natural food stores and will last. One fruit-based ingredient or a commercial moisturizer with 20+ ingredients: it's our choice to make.

Chapter Four
Removing Unnecessary Toxins From Your Home

Perhaps the easiest way to reduce toxic exposure is by removing the harsh chemical cleaners from your home. This takes very little effort and will end up costing you less in the long run.

I personally try to avoid walking down the "cleaning aides" aisle of any supermarket or box store because I find the mixture of all those smells nauseating. So why are we led to believe that we need one toxic cleaner for the laundry, another for the bath, one for kitchen surfaces and another for windows? It's because they are cheap to make and offer a high profit margin for chemical manufacturers.

Removing every germ from our living space should not be our goal. Our idea of hygiene has evolved into some sort of twisted chemical protection insanity. It has been suggested that by stripping all surfaces clean of every possible sign of bacteria, we are doing two things: first we are creating an environment in which super bacteria can evolve. Secondly, we are desensitizing our immune system to the rest of the world. If we are never exposed to germs in our house, what happens when you visit a friend who is natural minded and doesn't blast all available surfaces with toxins? Our bodies were built to handle most bacteria, good and bad, and by living a healthy existence with organic foods, exercise, love and low stress we increase our body's effectiveness in dealing with bacteria.

Even the FDA recognizes that antibacterial products are no more effective than using regular soap and water (Stromberg, 2014). Triclosan, the active ingredient in most antibacterial products, has not only been linked to hormonal disruption in laboratory animals and increased chances of developing allergies, but it also poses serious health risks to humans and the environment. Imagine how much of this stuff has been rubbed on your hands and washed down your sinks and drains.

Purchasing new products for the home can also expose us to harsh chemicals. Whenever we buy new clothing, bedding, mattresses and other products, we are likely breathing in toxic chemicals. New clothing and bedding are routinely sprayed with formaldehyde to preserve the material and prevent mildew. Flame retardants, used in the U.S. on furniture, car seats and infant bedding, and which are now banned in most other countries, are linked with cancer and nervous disorders. Their residues are so prevalent, it would take another eBook to cover the dangers they pose. Polyurethane, found in new mattresses, is a petroleum-based substance that emits volatile organic compounds (VOC's). VOC levels are between two and five times higher inside your home than out *and* VOC's show up in the exhalations of patients with lung, bowel and liver disease.

**Holistic Strategies
For Limiting Toxins in the Home**

Switch to regular soap and water when washing hands

You can safely and easily ditch the triclosan-laced anti-bacterials and switch to bar soap. My favorite is an olive soap by Kiss My Face that has minimal ingredients and no added fragrance. It cleans well and lathers up nicely. There are also essential oil based antibacterial hand sprays that are gentle, non-toxic and fit easily into a purse or backpack. I always carry around a small bottle of *Thieves Antibacterial Spray* during the winter months. The name came from the thieves who robbed the bodies of those who died of the bubonic plague in the 14th century. They used this blend of essential oils with simple base ingredients to avoid contracting the plague, which wiped out between 30 and 60% of all Europeans. If it's good enough for the plague, I figure it will help ward off the latest virus that's circulating.

Use Essential Oils

Differing from 'flavored' or 'scented' oils, essential oils are 100% extractions from one plant, like lavender or tea tree. Essential oils are made by steam distilling a large quantity of an herb. The result is a highly aromatic and potent vaporous liquid. These oils have many uses including natural cleaning products, herbal remedies, body care, aid in meditation, insect repellents and as natural perfume.

For home cleaning use, simply put 20-30 drops of the desired essential oil in a spray bottle, fill with water and voila - your homemade cleanser is ready to go. Just give a shake before use. It works great for kitchen surfaces, bathroom fixtures, windows, dusting and mopping. While most essential oils have antibacterial properties, I like to use lavender or tea tree essential oil. You could also use lemon, tangerine, eucalyptus or any other scent you like, or even a combination. My sister makes a great spray for bathroom 'odors' with a blend of grapefruit and tangerine essential oils with water. Refer to this table of essential oil properties to find the most potent antibacterials, antifungals, etc.

Though some people recommend taking diluted essential oils internally for health reasons, I do not recommend ingesting essential oils. They have many uses but I feel they are too strong for internal use. Using them for home cleaning is not only safe and effective, but it also reduces allergic reactions and respiratory problems in your home by eliminating toxic store brands. In fact, many essential oils act specifically on these symptoms. When purchasing essential oils, which can be bought online or in natural food markets and many grocery stores (if they have a 'natural' section), make sure you buy 100% Pure Essential Oils. That way, you are getting just the essential oil of that one plant, and no additives.

Try Baking Soda
Baking soda can you give you that texture you need for cleaning bathroom 'accessories' and also is great to flush down the toilet (and sinks, too) to enhance the workings of your septic system, if you live in a rural area. I also use it as laundry soap (1 cup per large load) and clothes come out smelling fresh and clean with no chemical overtones. If you're doing a dark load, mix the baking soda in the water first before adding clothes and use a little less.

Other Great Natural Cleaners

White vinegar As an all-around handy cleaner, white vinegar works well in cleaning floors, windows, stainless steel appliances and wood surfaces.

Hydrogen Peroxide A non-toxic bleaching agent, hydrogen peroxide can be used as a laundry whitener and stain remover.

Dr. Bonner's Pure Castile Liquid Soap This can be bought in bulk and diluted and added to your soap dispensers for the bathroom or kitchen. It also can be used to wash dishes, shampoo your hair, and carry out any general household cleaning projects.

By using these natural, plant based products, you are not only reducing the toxicity in your home, but you are lowering the amount of chemicals going down your drains and into the ground or eventual water supply. You also save money by using just a few cleaning agents that can be bought in bulk.

Wash All New Clothing and Bedding Before Use - With Baking Soda
This is a good way to reduce the toxic intake of your family. If you haven't already started, it's easy, quick and you end up with clothes and sheets that smell fresh without chemical undertones.

Buy Used or Organic Clothes and Bedding
Organic materials feel good to the touch and are expensive to buy, but certainly offer another option for chemical free clothes and bedding. Many of us have already begun to focus on purchasing recycled

household items. By doing this you are decreasing the amounts of chemicals brought into your home while limiting the trash ending up in landfills.

Chapter Five
What's in the Water?

Sometimes, when living in a place like Maine, where you are surrounded by lakes, streams and rivers and where water (and snow!) is still plentiful, you tend to not be concerned with the water supply. But whether you live here, or in some other city or country, the amount and quality of water should be on everyone's mind. As parts of our world experience drought and increased population, more and more focus is brought to the topic of water safety and preservation.

There are several ways that water can be contaminated. High levels of coliforms (bacteria and microbes that originate in the digestive systems of mammals, and soils and plants) increase the chances of water borne diseases. The presence of fecal coliforms, such as E.Coli, will also raise dangerous possibilities. An over-acidic pH level affects the water quality and can cause heavy metals to leach into the water supply.

Water contaminants can affect public drinking water and rural wells. People most at risk for water contamination tend to live near industrial sites, like mining operations, factories and commercial farms. These locations may pose serious health risks due to runoffs laden with nitrates and volatile organic compounds (like benzene).

The quality of local septic systems and sewage infrastructure can also play a part in the healthiness of your water. There may also be specific chemicals that are found in the ground water in your geographic location, such as radium or arsenic.

Substances used to treat public water include disinfectants such as Chlorine and Ozone, coagulants including iron and aluminum salts, pH adjustors like sodium hydroxide, and fluoridation chemicals. As you can see, there are far too many toxic possibilities in our drinking water alone.

Holistic Strategies
For Maximizing Water Quality

Test Your Water Regularly
About 85% of Americans have water piped into homes that is chemically treated and regulated by the Environmental Protection Agency (EPA). In rural areas, the remaining 15% have well water that must be tested and dealt with by the property owner.

The first step in securing clean water is creating an awareness of what's in your water. If you have city water and live in the U.S., then you can check the EPA's website here to review your local water quality reports.

For those with well water, you can easily get your water tested. Check your county or state government page for water quality and they will list certified water testing labs in your area. The state of Maine has a link on their website here that gives specific information on rural watersheds, approved water testing companies and information about what do to when a test comes back and what should cause concern. To have your well water or city water tested personally, it is a small fee for the testing kit (usually under $20.00) and many local governments have people in place that can support you in interpreting the test results.

Filter Your Drinking Water
To my knowledge, the best system of water filtration in homes is a solid block carbon filter. Though it may initially seem cost inhibitive (several hundred dollars) and can take up a lot of counter space, it is currently the most effective filtration system and removes more contaminants than the other choices (such as water pitcher filters, reverse osmosis systems and personal UV and solar water purifiers). While all filters will eliminate some compounds, the solid block carbon system appears to filter out the most.

Eat More Organic Raw Fruits
This may seem odd, but a body that receives abundant juicy fruits will need to drink less water than a body that is consuming only cooked foods (where the water is cooked out in almost all examples). Raw plants have a higher water content, leaving you less thirsty and contributing fiber, vitamins and minerals.

Tips for Maintaining a Safe Well
Testing is the first step, and can be done simply and cost effectively using links in the previous section. An annual or bi-annual schedule of testing will ensure your water is suitable for drinking.

The other important key is to be aware of what's going in the ground in your area, and controlling it whenever possible. You may not be able to change the fact that your home is near an industrial complex or a large farm, but you can make sure the septic system has been updated or checked. Choices may be made about what's sprayed on your lawn and garden and what goes down the drains of your home. If you have a well, whatever is poured into ground or into your septic and drainage system can end up in your drinking water.

Chelation Therapy With Cilantro
Cilantro is a naturally chelating herb, meaning it removes toxic metals from your bodily tissues. To undergo chelation therapy, simply incorporate a handful of fresh Cilantro into a daily meal for two or three weeks (check with your healthcare practitioner before undergoing chelation therapy). Cilantro is also a good source of iron, magnesium and manganese; is high in Vitamins K, C and A; and is full of phytonutrients like quercetin and camphor. My favorite way to eat cilantro is in a salsa but it's also great mixed with avocado and limejuice or added to any soup, pasta, stir-fry or pesto.

Chapter Six
Clearing Up The Air

We often hear about problems with air pollution and we're trained to pay attention to air quality indexes before spending time outside. While fresh air is so important for humans and getting out in nature is certainly my favorite health strategy, even more important is the quality of air inside your home. Even for those of us who are living in relatively clean air climates and are getting a good amount of fresh air, the reality is that the majority of our time is spent inside. It just makes sense to focus on indoor air solutions.

Holistic Strategies
For Improving Indoor Air Quality

Indoor Plants
Just as the trees absorb and utilize the carbon dioxide we exhale when outdoors, having indoor plants can also help absorb dirty air. Succulents, herbs, ferns and spider plants all have plentiful greens and are easy to keep as a potted plant.

Get Fresh Air Inside
In Maine, the heat is on about 8 or 9 months a year, making the air extremely dry and, depending on what type of heat is being used, the air quality can be quite low. The air can be freshened in your home by opening windows in a few places to ensure a cross breeze. Even if it's freezing out, 10-15 minutes per day of open windows is not going to

substantially raise your fuel cost and will help cleanse the inside air.

Trickle Ventilation Systems
In the city and other places where opening windows may not necessarily improve the air in your home, a *Trickle Ventilation System* can be used. It's basically a small filtered screen that fits right into your window and catches the air before it enters your house.

Air Conditioners
In my neck of the woods, most people do not have AC because it's never hot for very long. But whether you live in the boondocks like me, or in a suburban or metropolitan area, air conditioning helps to remove moisture and water-soluble pollutants from the air. A High Efficiency Particulate Air Filter (HEPA) can be installed in the AC unit offering a higher level of clean air for the home.

Ionizers
One of my children, who has asthma symptoms during the winter when he gets a bad cold, showed marked improvement once I put an Ionizer in his room. It was suggested to me that I run it during the day, and not at night during his sleep. There is a concern of ozone emissions but by having the ionizer do its job of attracting airborne particles during the day, we noticed less asthmatic symptoms in general. Because we do use wood heat as one of our heating options, indoor air quality is extremely important. It's easy to grasp that the wood heat air is dirtier because in the winter there is more dust, and screens on the windows that I keep open (the

loft upstairs gets too hot) need cleaning every few weeks; you can see the brown dust that the woodstove creates.

(As a quick aside, during the winter it is also essential to keep hydrated with the constant indoor heat. I always use humidifiers in the kids' rooms at night. Cleaning the humidifier with baking soda each week is needed, otherwise mildew will build up on the inner workings. Conversely, in humid conditions, a de-humidifier may be used to keep water borne particles to a minimum.)

Essential Oils
There are several ways to use 100% pure essential oils for respiratory aromatherapy in the home. I often will put a few drops on the pillow of a child with a cold and I sometimes will add some to the humidifier. You can buy infusers for about $20 and they work well, but you don't need one to enjoy the medicinal properties of essential oils. Eucalyptus and Peppermint essential oils are both perfect for respiratory ailments and for soothing and strengthening the lungs. Eucalyptus essential oil has anti-inflammatory, decongestant, expectorant and antibacterial properties, just to name a few. Peppermint essential oil is an expectorant, a sedative, a stomachic and an analgesic (pain reliever). They can be used separately or in combination.

Chapter Seven
Internal Poisoning:
Releasing Toxic Emotions

Anyone that has tried to improve their health by incorporating aerobic exercise, weight lifting, stretching and a cleaner diet, knows that these methods alone cannot ensure optimal health. It's a puzzle that needs all its pieces.

Inner strength, while it can certainly be enhanced by a physically stronger body and the accompanying endorphins it receives, cannot be sustained while regularly receiving negative emotional signals from others in our lives, from ourselves, or from society at large. Many of the signals come from frustration and stress related to social requirements that, however embedded in our world, often make no sense.

Other times, we live our lives without ever learning to deal with negative emotions; allowing them to bottle up and cause toxicity. In the fast paced, materialistic society in which we live, emotions are all too often swept to the side as we are trained and encouraged to 'grin and bear it'.

A build-up of toxic emotions commonly resurfaces in the form of anxiety, displaced anger or fear, and insomnia. Maybe you've experienced an outburst of anger (this isn't *like* you) or the strong and sudden feeling of being completely overwhelmed for no concrete reason. When these feelings do resurface and go untended, the health risks only multiply.

Long term stress like this can directly suppress the immune system, increase the chances of heart disease, and cause adrenal fatigue leading to further health challenges.

Simple strategies here can make a huge difference and can be learned and practiced by anyone. Some folks may find that having a counselor is helpful to help work through the pent up emotions and assist the healing process, while gently teaching you new methods of emotional response. The strategies described below have helped me tremendously during times of acute stress.

Holistic Strategies
For Releasing Emotional Toxicity

Mentality of Gratitude

We hear so many messages on social media, TV, everywhere: how to look, who to like, what to say, what political party to join, what to eat, etc., etc. Repeated messages suggesting what we SHOULD be doing and buying have been relayed through our heads and have saturated our social circles. These messages try to convince us that we are not whole until we have done or bought what they have said, setting us up for feelings of inadequacy and stress.

It helps to stop, take a minute, and visualize ten things you are grateful for in your present moment. I love this exercise because once I start, I can never stop at just ten. This little task can flip your mindset very quickly. Practicing it on a regular basis will cause you to be creative and get connected with things for which you're thankful, but hadn't thought of otherwise. On a really challenging or stressful day, my list might look like this: I am grateful for a roof over my head, running water, the love of my family, my children's smiles, the ability to read, jokes, soft cotton clothing, fresh fruit to eat, a cup of herbal tea whenever I want it, music, and on and on. Repeated on a regular basis, the practice teaches you to focus on all the good things in your life, instead of getting wrapped up in all its problems.

Laughter

If anything feels better, I can't think of it. There's so much humor in life and many of the stressful situations we face are actually quite funny if we can get out of our heads and relax a bit. The old saying, "laughter is the best medicine" is actually true. Laughing causes muscles throughout our bodies to stretch; quickens our pulse, increases oxygenation to our cells; enhances our immune response; stabilizes blood sugar levels; improves sleep patterns; and can decrease levels of chronic pain.

Spending time with your favorite funny friends and family members makes a great way to relax and balance negative stimulation with positive reinforcement. Luckily we live in an age where whatever brand of comedy that makes you laugh is readily available online. I'm so lucky to have family members that crack me up all the time, and as a mom, finding humor in daily life makes the world so much happier for all of us. (My goofy comedy online habit is Netflix' Parks and Recreation.)

Recognition and Processing Through Art Therapy
As negative emotions face us, instead of stuffing them down because they are too difficult to face, or because we are programmed to just ignore them and carry on, spending some time with that emotion and dealing with it in that moment can process that negative feeling and bring closure.

There are several ways to do this. My favorite is art therapy, which to me can mean writing or drawing. But it can be whatever art form relates to you; dancing, singing, whittling or any other creative form. The simple steps to this process include:

1.Let yourself feel the feeling, let it flow through while you recognize and name it (like, "I'm angry").

2.While thinking about this emotion, create something that helps you explain the feelings you are having (I write out all my thoughts about it).
3.Relax by deep breathing, exercising, walking, listening to music or talking a bath.

Here's what it looks like when I employ this method: I'm wicked pissed about something. I recognize my own anger and begin to write down feverishly. I actually have a password-protected file on my pc called, "Toxins". At first my writing might be full of expletives but as I go along, my whole body relaxes, my writing becomes more fluid and I start to see the many sides of the situation. The process relaxes me and I usually finish with some deep breaths.

Essential Oils For Assisting Emotional Release
100% pure essential oils may be used to aid the releasing of specific toxic emotions. For anger and general feelings of being overwhelmed, Roman Chamomile essential oil assists in encouraging a stronger emotional awareness and recognition. Thinking about the emotion while breathing in the aroma of a few drops of the oil sprinkled on a washcloth, in your bath, or in an infuser, gently helps you release negativity. Other essential oils that may be used include Rose for sadness, Lavender for fear, Frankincense for frustration, Peppermint for disappointment, Lemongrass for self hatred, and many others. This therapy can be combined with any of the above-mentioned strategies in this chapter. Refer to Chapter 4 for information about ways to use essential oils.

Chapter Eight
Workplace Toxicity: Minimizing Your Exposure

I'm going to be straight with you here. I had spent a lot of time writing this chapter with a clear picture in my head that the electromagnetic fields emitted by wifi and cell phone usage could be harmful to our health. I did some initial research, outlined and wrote the chapter with that viewpoint in mind, finding plenty of online sources to support my opinion. During the writing process I always had the nagging feeling that I didn't have enough evidence to support this view.

During my last edits, I went through all the sources I had referenced in the book and started doing some double-checking. When I got to this chapter, as much as I hated to because of my veganism, I began to delve deep and read the animal studies that had been done to find negative health consequences of low frequency emf's. Many studies were done but no conclusive evidence was shown.

I thought about deleting the chapter completely but something made me want to stay with it. I know that keeping my laptop on my lap makes me feel a burning sensation on my legs and I know that if I use the touchpad as opposed to the mouse when word processing on my laptop, my fingers get a little numb after a while. I know that if I work on the computer right before bed it's more difficult to fall asleep than if I go screen-free for the few hours leading up to bedtime. I also know that sitting in place staring into one spot does not feel as good as walking, or other movements. Lastly, there are just too many reports, blog posts and opinions of people all across Internet to completely sweep all concern under the carpet.

So I'm going to go out on a limb here and keep my chapter in. I'll give suggestions that may possibly, yet without evidence, protect against over exposure to emf's.

Holistic Strategies
For Over Exposure To EMF's

Put Distance Between You and Your Devices
It is commonly accepted that the more distance between you and the source of EMF's, the lower the frequency. I think a good general guideline for cell phones use is to keep them out of your pocket and off your body, at least for extended durations. Do not keep devices under your pillow, or even hold your cell phone to your ear for a long time.

My gut tells me to keep as much distance between our bodies and the router or hot spot as is practical. What both sides of the argument agree upon is that distance between you and your devices reduces the levels of radiofrequency electromagnetic radiation.

Turn Off Router/Disable Wifi When Not in Use
Most laptops, desktops and other devices have an on/off switch for wireless connections. Some routers and modems also have a switch and others can be shut off using the wireless options menus on your computer. Turn them all off at night and when not in use. I know this sounds unrealistic and I'm

still trying to incorporate this into my own home (which is my workplace).

Melatonin for Insomnia
Because the light from our devices' screens can inhibit your body's nightly release of the hormone, Melatonin, which signals our bodies for sleep readiness, watching a screen during the hours leading up to sleep time can cause insomnia. Working during the nighttime hours on a computer regularly can, over time, lead to other health problems. Supplementing with Melatonin, under your health care practitioner's guidance, has been shown to help restore sleep patterns. You could also limit your screen time after 6pm or at least have a few hours of non-screen time before bed. I have also found that changing the default screen settings to darker colors (mine is light gray-green), especially for long-term word processing and reading, feels better on my eyes.

Yarrow Herb For Absorbance
I have to be honest and say there is zero research about Yarrow absorbing electromagnetic interference. But there are a lot of folk herbal theories. Personally, I have noticed that this wild plant seems to have it's own electromagnetic field. I have taken many pictures of yarrow and I can never get a truly clear shot - it's like it has an aura. Folk medicine suggests that a Yarrow Flower Essence be prescribed for those who are overly sensitive to their environment. I also once met a homeopathic doctor who had a vase of dried Yarrow flowers directly next to her pc, because, as she put it, it reduced her electromagnetic exposure. As an herbalist I want to say this will work in reducing

environmental toxins but it's effectiveness has not been scientifically proven by any stretch. I feel it definitely deserves further study.

Conclusion
Many Options For Making A Difference

In writing this book, I did not intend to suggest that everybody should all at once give up their favorite foods, electronic devices, prescriptions and all other sources of chemical exposure! It is unrealistic to think that so much change could happen overnight and it would undoubtedly cause undue stress to even attempt it. I wrote this book for people wanting to reduce their personal toxic load - to give them *many* options for eliminating dangers so they may easily improve their health by making a few common sense choices. By adopting a couple of the strategies outlined in this book, you are already making a difference.

While our world may be full of the threat of toxic exposure, it is also filled with hope. Those of us who have begun our journey to better health have the opportunity to learn more, live better and teach others.

Find more books by Mary Thibodeau under that author name at Amazon.com Kindle Store. Thank you!

References:

Total Number of Doctors in Medicine In The U.S. from 1949 to 2012. (2015). Retrieved on 8/8/2015 from http://www.statista.com/statistics/186260/total-doctors-of-medicine-in-the-us-since-1949/

Historical Population. (2015). Retrieved on 8/13/2015 from https://en.wikipedia.org/wiki/Demographic_history_of_the_U nited_States#Historical_population

Cancer And Your Environment. (2012). Retrieved on 8/11/2015 from http://www.idph.state.il.us/cancer/factsheets/cancer.htm

What Is The Meaning Of "Natural" On The Label Of Food. (2015). Retrieved on 8/11/2015 from http://www.fda.gov/aboutfda/transparency/basics/ucm214868. htm

H.R. 2044 113th Congress 1st Session. (2013). Retrieved on 8/11/2015 from http://www.gpo.gov/fdsys/pkg/BILLS-113hr2044ih/html/BILLS-113hr2044ih.htm

Pesticides Industry Sales and Usage. (2007). Retrieved on 8/11/2015 from http://www.epa.gov/opp00001/pestsales/07pestsales/market_e stimates2007.pdf

2014 Maine Wild Blueberry Pesticide Chart. (2014). Retrieved on 8/15/2015 from http://umaine.edu/blueberries/files/2010/05/2014-ME-Wild-Blueberry-Pesticide-Chart-Insecticides_Revised-on-5-7-2014.pdf

Mosbergen, D. (2014). Organic Food Has More Antioxidants; Less Pesticide Residue, Study. Retrieved on 8/20/2015 from http://www.huffingtonpost.com/2014/07/12/organic-food-study_n_5579174.html

The "Dirty Dozen". (2015). Retrieved on 8/20/2015 from

http://www.organic.org/articles/showarticle/article-214

Company Fact Sheet. (2015). Retrieved on 8/20/2015 from http://www.merck.com/about/our-history/facts/home.html

Swanson, Ana. (2015). Big Pharmaceuticals Companies Are Spending Far More Money On Marketing Than Research. Retrieved on 8/21/2015 from http://www.washingtonpost.com/blogs/wonkblog/wp/2015/02/11/big-pharmaceutical-companies-are-spending-far-more-on-marketing-than-research/

Skin Deep Product And Ingredient Databases. (2015). Retrieved on 8/21/2015 from http://www.ewg.org/skindeep/site/about.php

Why This Matters: Cosmetics And Your Health. (2011). Retrieved on 8/21/2015 from http://www.ewg.org/skindeep/2011/04/12/why-this-matters/

Stromberg, J. (2014). Five Reasons Why You Should Probably Stop Using Antibacterial Soap. Retrieved on 8/22/2015 from http://www.smithsonianmag.com/science-nature/five-reasons-why-you-should-probably-stop-using-antibacterial-soap-180948078/?no-ist

www.ingramcontent.com/pod-product-compliance
Lightning Source LLC
Chambersburg PA
CBHW071219280526
45787CB00002B/733